STRETCHING EXERCISES FOR SENIORS

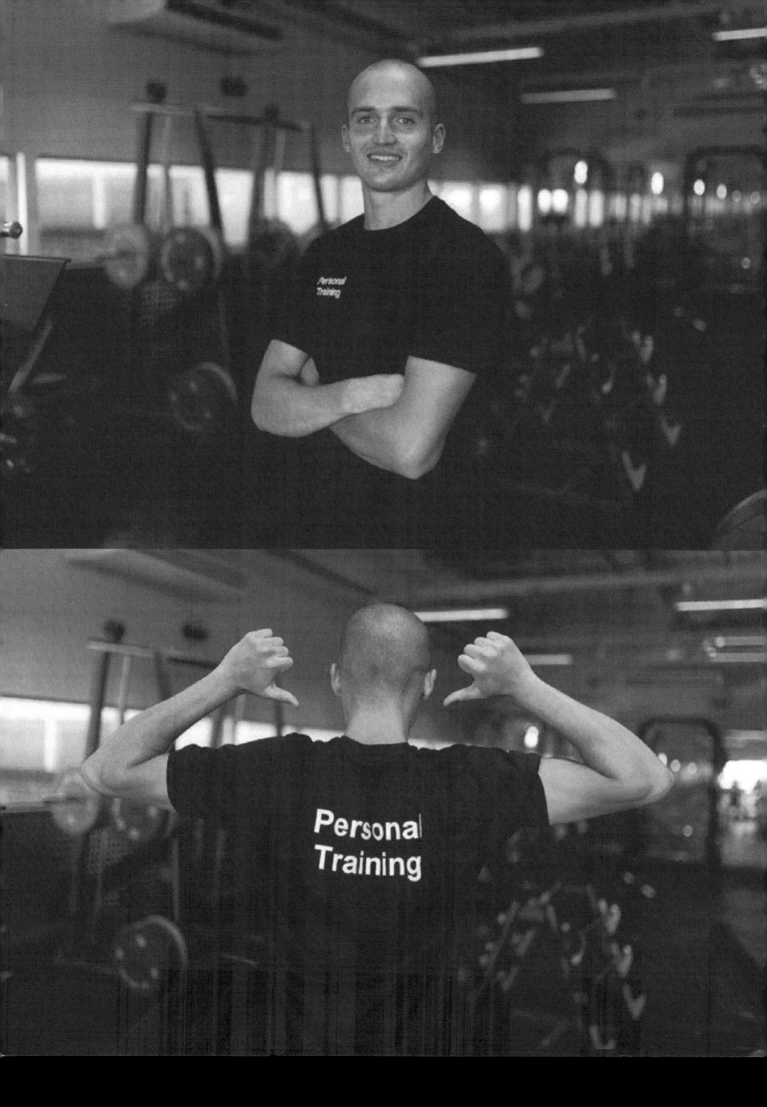

Instructed by a Certified Personal Trainer

Disclaimer

The information provided in this book is intended for educational and informational purposes only. It is not a substitute for professional medical advice, diagnosis, or treatment. Always seek the advice of yourphysician or other qualified healthcare provider before starting any new fitness program or making any changes to an existing one. The author and publisher of this book are not responsible for any injury or health problems that may result from the use of the information in this book.

CONTENTS

CHAIR ASSISTED

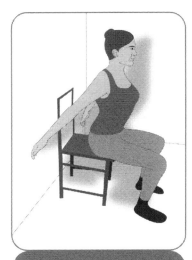

Shoulder Stretch

Pag 07

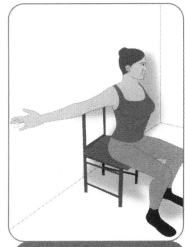

Shoulder Stretch (Variation)

Pag 09

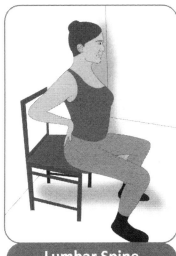

Lumbar Spine Stretch

Pag 11

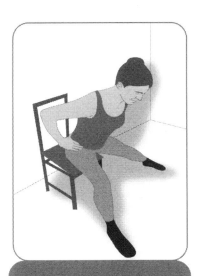

Groin Stretch

Pag 13

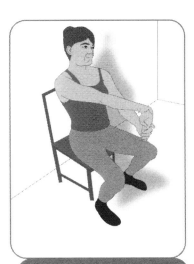

Wrist Flexion Stretch

Pag 15

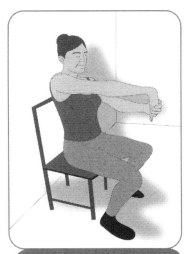

Wrist Extension Stretch

Pag 17

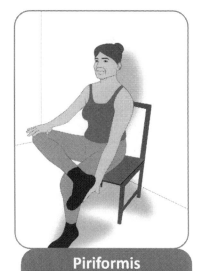

Piriformis Stretch

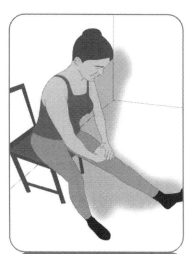

Calf And Hamstring Stretch

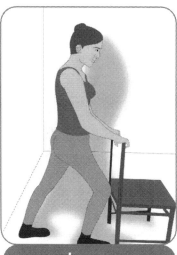

Lower Body Stretch

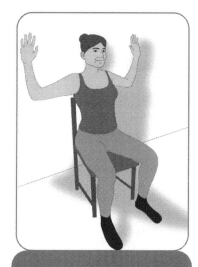

Goal Post Stretch

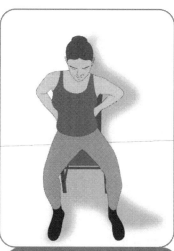

Seated Hip Circle

FLOOR EXERCISES

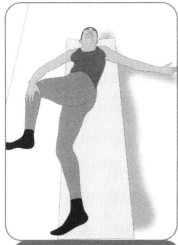

Lumbar Rotation Stretch

Pag 29

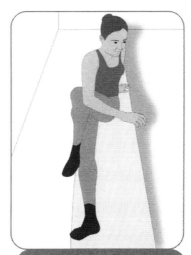

Seated Spine Stretch

Pag 31

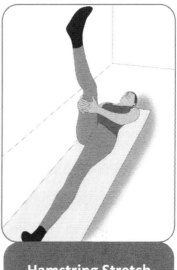

Hamstring Stretch

Pag 33

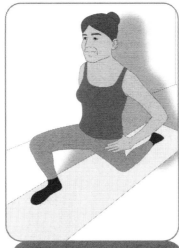

Hip Flexor Stretch

Pag 35

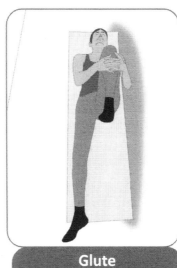

Glute Stretch

Pag 37

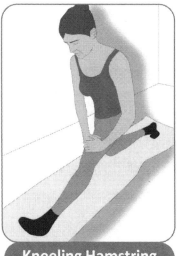

Kneeling Hamstring Stretch

Pag 39

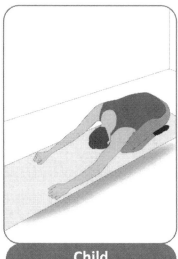

Child Pose Stretch

Pag 41

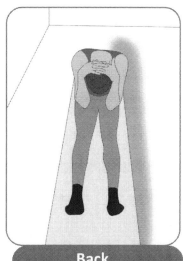

Back Extension Stretch

Pag 43

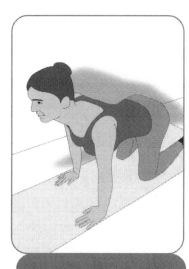

Cat Cow Stretch

Pag 45

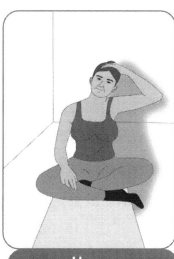

Upper Trap Release

Pag 47

STANDING EXERCISES

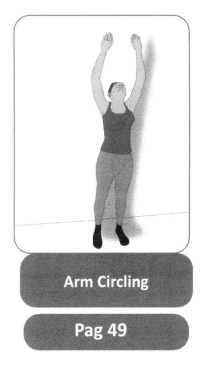

Arm Circling

Pag 49

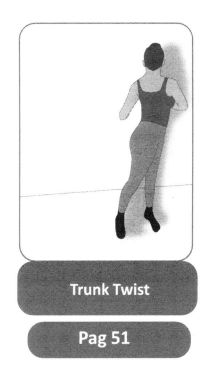

Trunk Twist

Pag 51

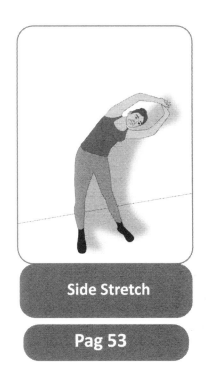

Side Stretch

Pag 53

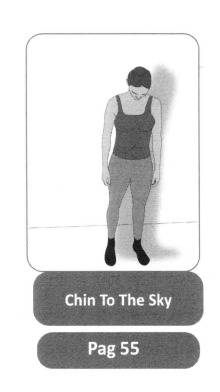

Chin To The Sky

Pag 55

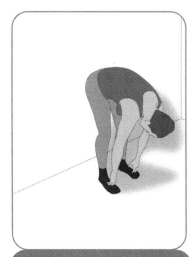

Toe Touch +
Arm Raise

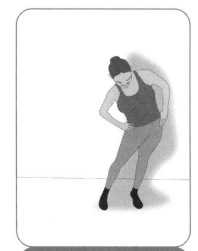

Hip Circle

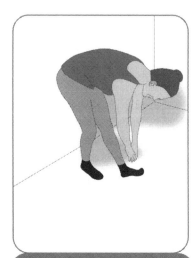

Hamstring
Stretch

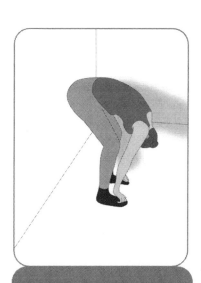

Toe Touch

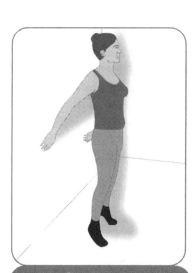

Heel Raises + Arm
Swing

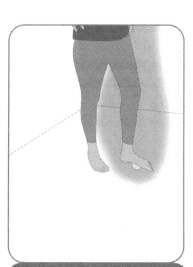

Bonus Exercise:
Plantar Fascia Roll

INTRODUCTION

The old saying "use it or lose it" applies perfectly here!

Due to sedentary lifestyles and a high level of stress, we tend to have more joint pain and muscle ache than ever before. Our muscles are always tense, and we don't feel well.

With all this tension and stress we face on a daily basis, it is inevitable that over time, they will translate into physical tension, leading to pain and discomfort in our neck, back, shoulders, hips, and any muscles we have, without any clear reason.

Ideally, for every 8 hours of sitting you should be moving your body for an hour…

What if you can just spend a few minutes per day to reverse the effect of the modern lifestyle? and what if you are not even going to suffer or make a crazy effort to achieve that?

The book focuses on helping you feel better and less stiff, so that when stress arises, you can go to your "safe space" where you can stretch and relax your body.

In today's society, sitting is the new smoking, and in order to feel good and stay healthy, it is essential to stretch and move on a daily basis.

If you relax your body, your mind will follow!

TIPS TO STAY CONSISTENT AND MAINTAIN MOTIVATION DURING THE PROGRAM

I am sure now you have plenty of motivation and you're looking forward to starting and finding out what the exercises and routine are (also, I have a feeling you might skip this part and go straight to the exercises.) However, if you are reading this, I am confident these tips will greatly benefit you in staying consistent with the month-long plan even on days when you may not feel like exercising.

Here are four methods:

Note: You do not need to use all of them, maybe even one can make a difference for you to stay consstent.

- **Future Visualization.**

I would encourage you to imagine how you would look, feel, and be in a month from now if you exercise consistently, even on days when you're not up to it. This visualization can be a powerful motivator. You might picture yourselves with better posture, increased vitality, reduced joint pain, or even fitting into an outfit you love. Use your goal as fuel here!

- **Social Connections**

Having an accountability partner can go a long way! The benefits of sharing your goals with someone and what you want to achieve will give you a sense of responsibility, increased willpower, and can also make your journey more fun!

- **Set Achievable Goals and Celebrate Milestones**

Breaking down the fitness journey into smaller, manageable goals can make the process less daunting. Perhaps the initial goal would be to complete the first session, then the first week (which includes only three workouts, making it very manageable), and gradually increasing the challenge over time. Celebrating each achieved milestone, no matter how small, can foster a sense of accomplishment and motivation to keep going. Imagine how good you will feel when you're doing five sessions per week in week 3 or 4.

- **Integrate Variety and Keep it Fun**

Doing the same routine every day can become monotonous. This is why I've come up with these routines where everyday you'll do different exercises to keep it enjoyable and fun!

Another option is to do them at different times throughout the day. Try doing them as soon as you wake up, before lunch, in the afternoon and before going to sleep... Figure out what works best for you, and then stick with it!

These methods, or at least one of them, can help you stay motivated and make regular exercise a consistent part of your lifestyle.

COMMON MISTAKES FOR STRETCHING EXERCISES

- *Breathing*: This is a crucial point and I want to make it very very clear before starting. Do not be tense or hold your breath. Always do long exhales and do your very best to relax all parts of your body when stretching, especially the targeted muscle.

  Try to inhale through your nose and exhale through your mouth, emptying your lungs.

  Ps: In every stretch I write how long it's optimal and recommended to hold it. However, if instead of counting the seconds you prefer to count your breath, feel free to do so. Many people prefer it this way.

  In that case, hold each stretch between **3 breaths (roughly 10"-15") and 5 breaths (20"- 30")**.

Ps: In the case of an injury, you should not stretch for 72 hours after the injury has occurred

- **Neglecting to Warm Up:** Obviously, as this routine is just stretching (and it does nor include heavy or intense exercises), you won't need to run a mile or do any intense activity. However, I would highly recommend to even just go for a walk and do some light movement for 5-10 minutes before doing the stretches. This will enhance your range of motion when stretching as the muscles will be already warm and ready to be stretched effectively!

Ps: In the case of an injury, you should not stretch for 72 hours after the injury has occurred

- **Keep each stretch comfortable:** You have to push so that you will relax the muscle, but never make it painful or uncomfortable. The main benefits of stretching is doing a gentle workout to keep you mobile and less stiff, without causing soreness or pain that lasts for days.

Keep in mind that a long gentle 30'' stretch is way more effective to release muscle and joints than a 5'' intense stretch (that would actually be harmful at times).

Extra Notes Worth to Keep in Mind

- Stretch whenever you like. However, the best time to do that is either in the morning to start moving gently and wake up more focused and alert. On the other hand, stretching before going to sleep is very effective as it helps falling asleep faster and deeper.
- I suggest you do it with socks or barefoot if possible as it helps to promote a better blood flow and being more aware of your body. However, this is a simple recommendation that is not going to change the efficacy of the exercises.

Also, if you feel like some explanation are not esaustive, and you feel like you need some extra tips regarding your fitness, please do not hesitate to contact me either via email at avfitness99coaching@gmail.com or on Instagram at avfitness99

CHAIR ASSISTED

SHOULDER STRETCH

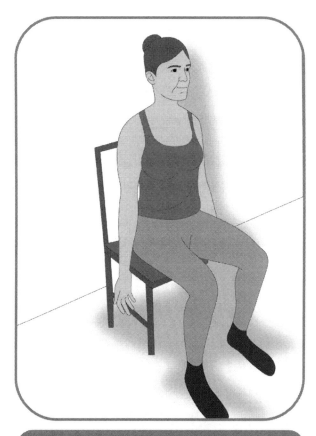

Step 1 - Starting Position with arms in line with your trunk

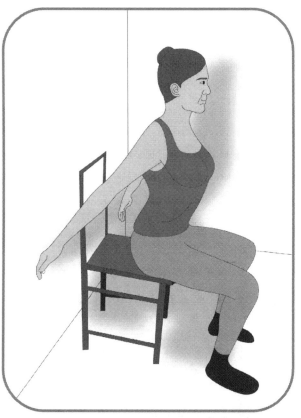

Step 2 – Bring arms back and hold for 20''. Then, release

How to do it:

1. Sit comfortably keeping your trunk up and tall - avoid touching the backrest - keep your arms straight next to your body with palms facing forward, as shown in Step 1.

2. From there, bring your arms back keeping them straight. As you do so, squeeze your shoulder blades together, open your chest and hold it for 20''. Keep looking in front of you.

3. Then, come back into the starting position and release the stretch. Keep breathing throughout the 20 seconds of stretch.

Note:

A very useful tip is that during the stretch you focus on keeping your chest open and high. This will ensure the front part of your shoulders are stretched effectively. I suggest you shake your arms after the stretch.

SHOULDER STRETCH
(Variation)

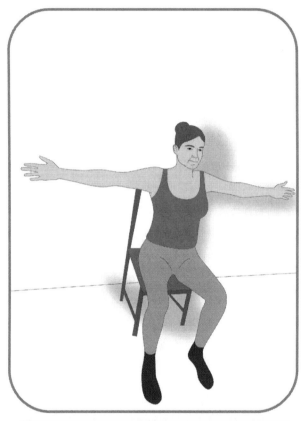

Step 1 - Starting Position with arms parallel to the floor

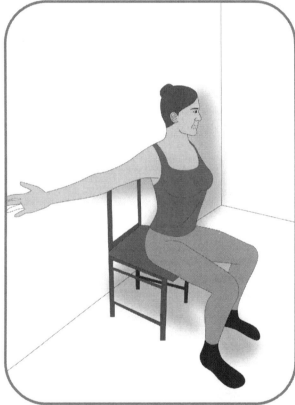

Step 2 - Bring arms back, keep chest up and stretch

How to do it:

1. Sit comfortably keeping your trunk up and tall keeping your arms open to the side parallel to the floor, as shown in Step 1.

2. From there, bring your arms back keeping them straight. As you do so squeeze your shoulder blades together keeping your chest open and hold it for 20'', as the variation in the previous page.

3. Then, come back into the starting position and release the stretch- shake your arms after it.

Note:

This will not only make sure that the front part of your shoulders are squeezed, but also your chest. As mentioned previously, I suggest shaking your arms after the stretch.

LUMBAR SPINE STRETCH

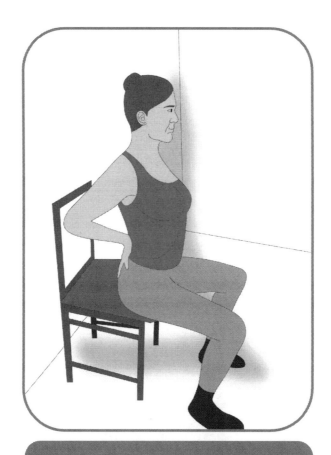

Hold it gently for 30", then release

How to do it:

1. Sit on a chair with a bit of distance from the backrest.

2. Place your hands on your lower back whilst sitting on a chair. Maintain your trunk straight.

3. Press with your hands on the side of the lower back and bring your chest up and forward so that to extend your spine, focusing on opening up the upper back area.

4. Hold that stretch for 30''. and then release.

Note:

In our daily life activities we spend so much time leaning forward and working the front side of the body, without really working and strengthening the lumbar spine. This can make it weak and stiff over time. Here is a simple yet effective stretch to counteract the modern lifestyle.

Also, you can perform the stretch in a standing position if you prefer.

GROIN STRETCH

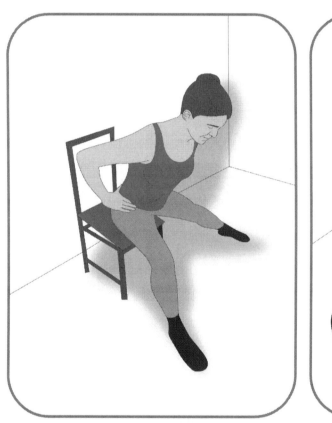

Stretch left groin gently for 20''

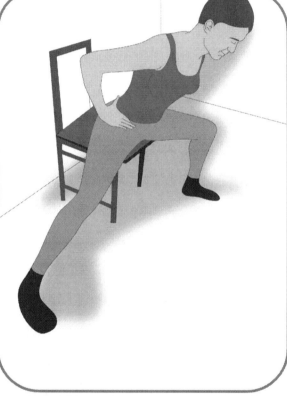

Then, stretch right groin for 20''

How to do it:

1. Sit on the brink of the chair and bring your left leg on the side keeping it straight. Keep your toes pointing forwards, as shown in the image.

2. The other leg slightly pointing on the side whilst keeping your knees bent at roughly 90°.

3. From there, lean forward slightly so that you will feel a stretch on the inner thigh of the straightened leg. Keep your chest up and back straight as you do so - keep hands on your waist.

4. Hold it for 20'' and then repeat it on the other side.

Note:

Often our groin can become tight due to lack of movements. This stretch will open them up. Remember to lean forward just as far as you feel comfortable, without exaggerating.

You can also do this stretch in a standing position, even though that would be more advanced and complicated.

WRIST FLEXION STRETCH

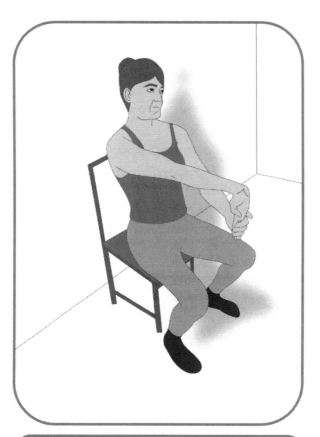

Stretch your wrist with the right palm facing forward - initially palm facing the ceiling, then flex your wrist and hold it for 10".

How to do it:

1. Sit and straighten the right arm in front of you with your palm facing the ceiling.

2. Grab the right fingers with your left hand and push the right fingers down.

3. You are going to feel a stretch in our right wrist. Hold it for 10'', and switch sides.

Note:

This is also great for preventing any injuries for your wrist including Carpal Tunnel. Some people when doing this stretch feel a muscle they did not even know they had! It's an effective and underrated stretch.

Before switching sides, I would suggest you shake your hands first.

WRIST EXTENSION STRETCH

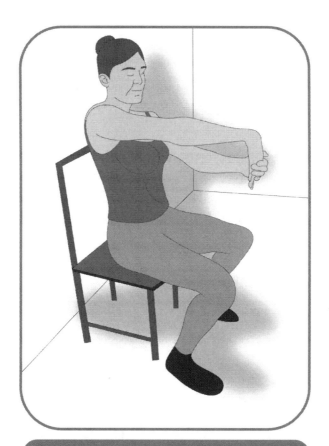

Stretch your wrist with palms
facing you - initially palm facing down

How to do it:

1. Sit and straighten the right arm in front of you with your palm facing down

2. Grab the right fingers with your left hand and push the right fingers down.

3. You are going to feel a stretch in your right wrist, especially the upper part. Hold it very gently for 10'', and switch sides.

Note:

Same as the previous stretch. It is going to work the muscles on the other side of the wrists.

As suggested previously, before switching sides I would suggest you to shake your hands first.

PIRIFORMIS STRETCH

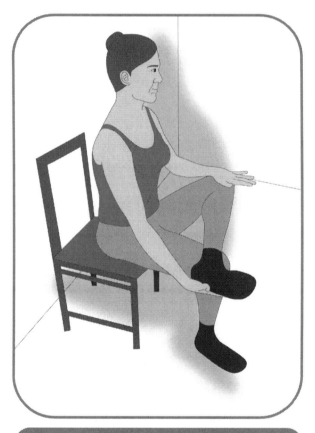

Stretch Left Glute

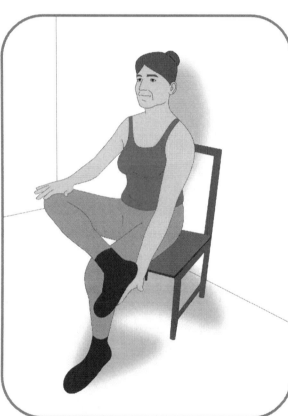

Stretch Right Glute

How to do it:

1. Sit up on the edge of a chair maintaining your back flat.

2. Now place your left foot on the right thigh, as shown in the image.

3. Then, place your left hand on the left knee and gently push it down.

4. At the same time place your right hand on your left foot, pulling it towards you, as shown in the image.

5. Hold the stretch for 10'', and then switch sides.

Note:

Keep your trunk straight nice and tall as you do the stretch so that you are not going to feel it on your glute but also on the hip area (the outer part). Remember to be gentle.

Also, it's quite common that one side is more mobile than the other. If that's the case spend an extra 5'' on the stiffer side, so that overtime it will catch up.

CALF AND HAMSTRING STRETCH

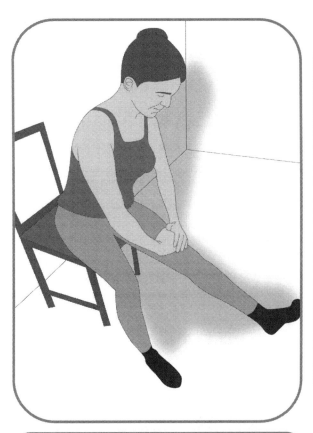

Stretch Left leg for 15" (Keep right leg bent).

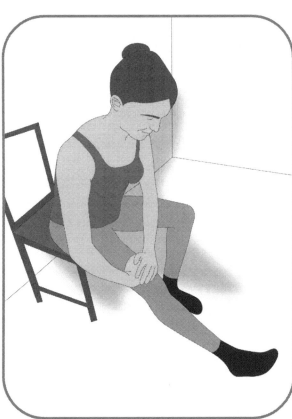

Then, do the other leg

How to do it:

1. Sit on the edge of the chair and bring your left leg straight in front of you with the heel touching the floor.

2. Whilst keeping your back straight, bring your hands together and as you lean with your body forward towards your foot, placing them on your left knee.

3. Place them on your shinbone if you do not feel any stretch placing them on your knee.

4. Hold the stretch for 15'', and then switch sides.

Note:

Do you know tight hamstrings can contribute to low back and hip pain? This stretching will not only improve your mobility, but also reduce and prevent joint aching.

To feel it more on your calves, flex your foot up with toes pointing toward you (as much as possible for you). This simple movement will work amazingly to stretch the muscle above your ankle, at the back of your lower leg.

LOWER BODY STRETCH

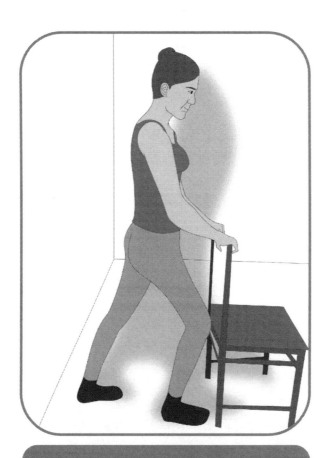

Stretch the left leg. Then, switch sides.

How to do it:

1. Stand behind a chair and bring one leg back as shown in the image. Keep both front and back legs straight.

2. Hold onto the chair with your hands and start bending your front knee forward whilst keeping the back leg straight (with heel on the floor). You are going to feel your hip flexor muscle and calf muscle of the back leg stretching gently.

3. Hold this position for 30'', and then repeat it on the other side.

Note:

This is very good especially if you sit for a prolonged period of time. Over time our hips suffer from this, so this nice stretch is what you need for reversing the negative effects of sitting.

When performing this exercise, remember to keep your trunk straight and do not bend forward.

The more you bring your back leg backward, the more you'll feel the stretch.

GOAL POST STRETCH

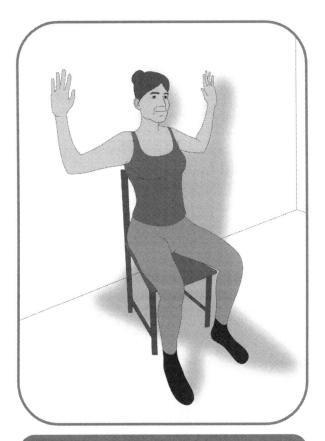

*Hold the position gently for 20'',
then release.*

How to do it:

1. Sit comfortably resting your back on a chair.

2. Lifting your arms parallel to the floor. Then, lift the forearm vertical to the floor, keeping your wrist straight.

3. From there, pinch your shoulder blades together, and feel your chest and front part of your shoulders opening up.

4. Hold the stretch for 20'' and then release.

Note:

This is one of the few stretches here that requires you also to contract some muscles - here are the upper back muscles. The benefits are immense for posture and shoulder health if you do this exercise correctly and consistently.

Remember to keep your neck relaxed.

SEATED HIP CIRCLE

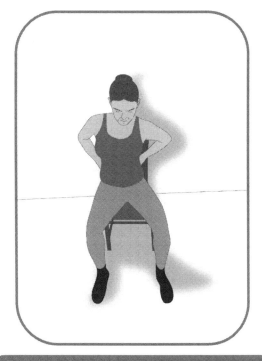

Gently move your hips towards the right side.

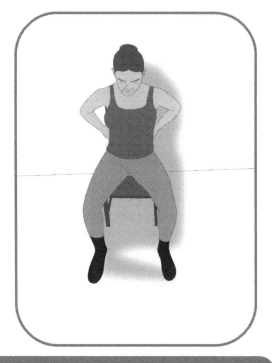

Then, move them forwards (gently, without forcing any movement)

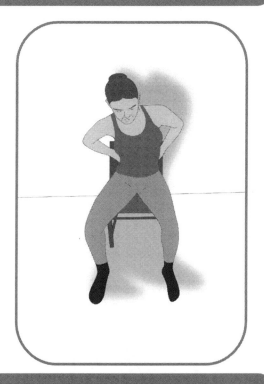

Then, move them towards the left side

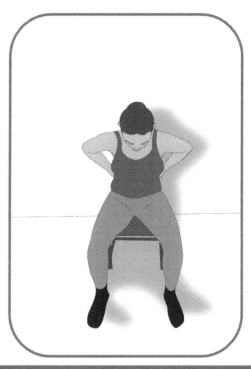

Lastly, move them backwards. Keep repeating the circle with your hips for the mentioned times.

How to do it:

1. Sit comfortably with feet hip width apart and hands behind your lower back. Feet planted on the floor.

2. From there, move your hips in a circle. Start gently in a clockwise motion. Do it 10 times.

3. Then, move them in the opposite direction (anticlockwise) for 10 times.

Note:

Very gentle exercise to loosen up your waist and get used to this movement. Make small circles first. Then, once you feel more comfortable you can make those circles bigger.

If it feels more comfortable you can position your hands on your waist (one the side, specifically) rather than your lower back.

Feel free to send a video of your execution at avfitness99coaching@gmail.com to make sure your technique is right, or to simply ask for more training tips.

As a more challenging alternative, perform Hip Circle in the Standing Exercises Section.

FLOOR EXERCISES

LUMBAR ROTATION
STRETCH

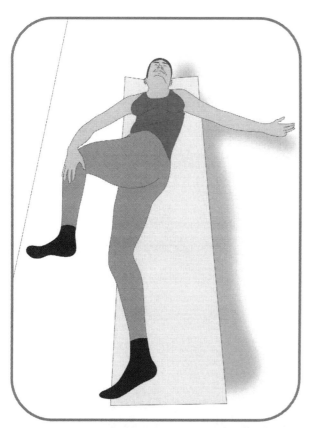

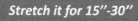

Stretch it for 15''-30''

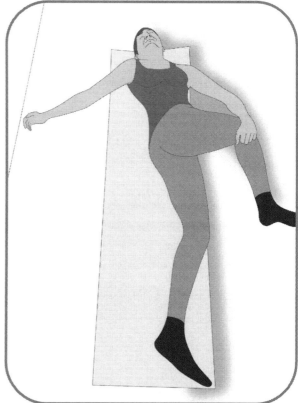

Then, repeat on the other side

How to do it:

1. Lay down with your back in contact with a mat.

2. Then, have your left knee bent, and with your right hand grab the outside of your left knee.

3. Pull the left leg over to the right side whilst keeping the bend at the knee.

4. Hold this position for 15-30''. Then, repeat it on the other side.

Note:

You will feel a stretch around your lower back and hip. Pull the leg to the side as you feel comfortable. Over time you will notice you can go deeper into the stretch.

SEATED SPINE STRETCH

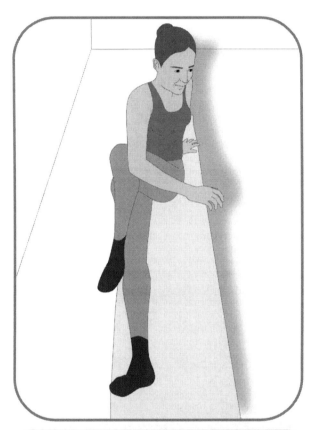

Stretch it on one side, bringing your left leg over the right one

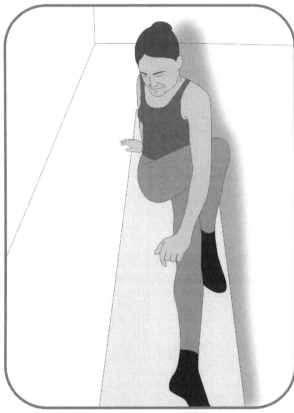

Then, do it on the other side

How to do it:

1. Sit on the floor. with legs straight in front of you.

2. Cross your left leg over your right one, and place your left foot on the floor.

3. Place your right elbow on the outside of your left knee. Also, place your left hand on the floor for support.

4. Slightly push with your right elbow the left leg towards the right side, and rotate your body towards the left side.

5. You will feel a stretch on your glutes and low back. Hold it for 20''. Then, come back into the starting position, and repeat on the other side.

Note:

Easy stretch that anyone can do regardless of the initial fitness level. If you are particularly stiff, simply crossing your leg over will make you feel a stretch already.

Also, rotate your body towards the opposite side as you feel comfortable.

One common mistake many people make when performing this stretch is to not keep their back straight. Keep it straight and tall, even when you rotate your trunk, to ensure maximal effectiveness.

HAMSTRING STRETCH

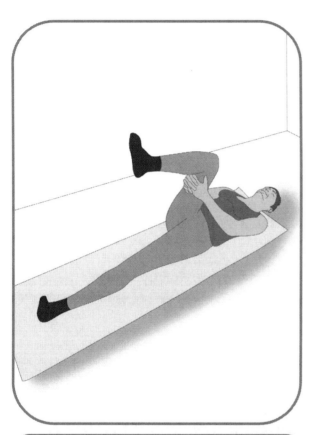

Step 1 - Lift one leg with knee bent

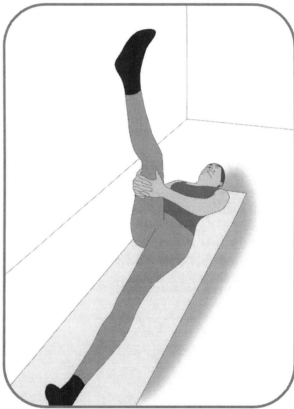

Step 2 - Extend the leg and stretch gently.
Then, repeat it with the other leg

How to do it:

1. Lay down with your back on the mat and lift one leg with your knees bent - and foot in the air. The other leg stays straight with the heel on the floor.

2. Grab the lifted leg with both hands just over the kneecap, on your thigh.

3. From there, extend that leg so that your sole is pointing at the ceiling.

4. Hold the stretch for 15''. Then, repeat on the other side.

Note:

You will feel a stretch on the hamstring muscles at the back of your thigh. You will definitely feel it close to the glute. Overtime, you will be able to extend and straighten your leg completely, you are also going to feel it closer to the calf muscle.

Remember to keep your head in contact with the floor. Some people tend to elevate it. This might cause neck pain and soreness around the upper back.

HIP FLEXOR STRETCH

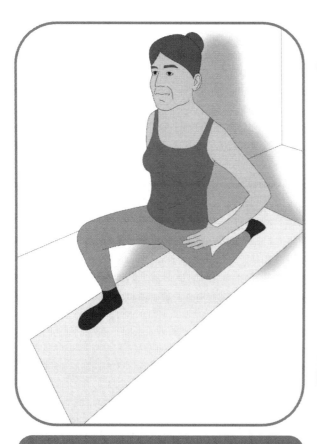

Stretch the left Hip Flexor

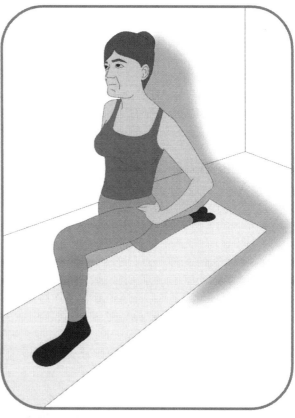

Then, repeat it on the other side holding gently the stretch for 15"

How to do it:

1. Place your left knee on the ground and take a lunge with your right leg, placing your right foot on the floor.

2. Keep your hands either on the side, your waist or on your right thigh.

3. Push your glute and hip forward whilst keeping your trunk upright. Feel the stretch on the left hip flexor (upper part of your thigh), and hold it for 15''.

4. Lastly, repeat it on the other side.

Note:

Oftentimes, low back pain is caused by tight hip flexor. Incorporating this stretch on your routine will prevent the likelihood of low back pain, or even letting it go away!

GLUTE STRETCH

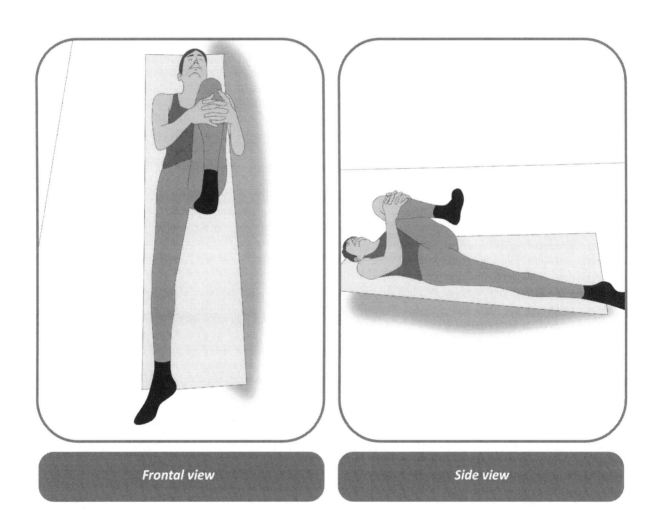

Frontal view

Side view

How to do it:

1. Lay on a mat extending your legs in front of you.

2. Bring your left knee towards your chest grabbing your shinbone with your hands (close to knee level).

3. Pull it towards your chest until you feel the stretch around your left hip. Hold it for 15'', and then repeat on the other side.

Note:

Also known as Piriformis Stretch, will help loosen up your glutes and the hips, making daily movements easier. We spend lots of time sitting nowadays, so stretching our hips is crucial to prevent mobility in the lower body.

KNEELING HAMSTRING STRETCH

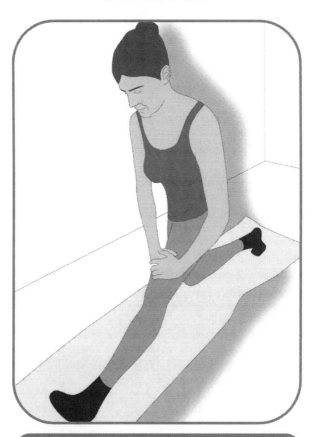

Hold the stretch for 15''-30''.
Then, switch sides.

How to do it:

1. Start with your right knee on the floor, and your left leg straight in front of you with only your left heel on the floor.

2. Then, lean forward with your trunk whilst keeping your left leg straight. Keep your hands on the front thigh.

3. Feel a stretch on your left hamstrings - back of your thigh - and hold the stretch from anywhere between 15'' and 30''.

4. Then, repeat it on the other side. So left knee on the floor, right leg straight in front of you, and lean forward.

Note:

I highly suggest you use a thick mat to do this exercise so that the knee on the floor does not have too much pressure on it.

Alternatively, if you cannot use a mat, place a pillow under the knee so that you avoid pain and discomfort.

A minority of people struggle with balance. If that's you, have a wall or a chair next to you so that you can hold it with one of your hands for safety.

CHILD POSE STRETCH

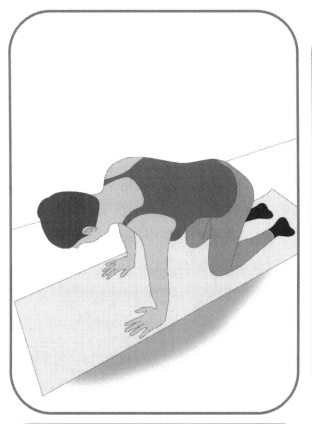

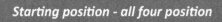

Starting position - all four position

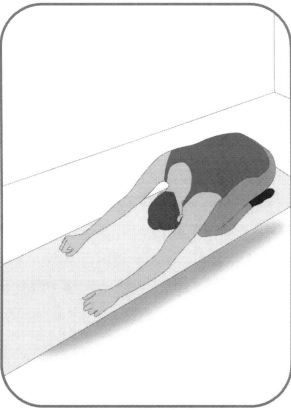

Stretching Position - Glutes and heels close to each other, stretch gently your back

How to do it:

1. Start in all four positions with knees under hips and hands under your shoulders.

2. Then, sit on your heels bringing your glutes back as close as possible to your feet. Keep your arms and back straight.

3. Hold that position for 15'', and then release, coming back into the starting position.

Note:

One of the best stretches to release low and upper back tension as well as improving posture and relax the whole body.

As an extra tip I suggest you tuck your chin so that you will release any pressure on your neck and upper traps.

BACK EXTENSION STRETCH

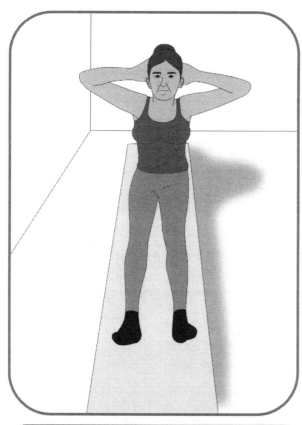

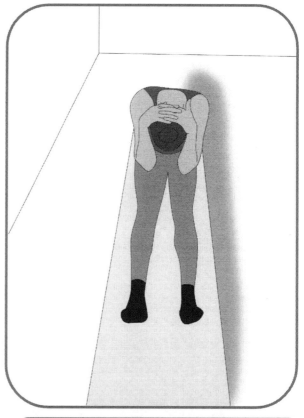

Starting Position - Sit on the floor with legs straight (minimal knee bent is ok) and trunk straight, parallel to the floor.

Bring elbows together, tuck your chin and fold forward gently to stretch your spine. Then, come back into the starting position.

How to do it:

1. Sitting on the floor with legs straight in front of you (minimal bend at the knees) is acceptable.

2. Now place your fingertips to the back of your head.

3. Fold forward bringing your elbows together. Also tuck your chin in,you are going to feel a stretch on your upper back. Hold it for 2''

4. Then, open your chest up looking at the ceiling. Separate your elbows and keep your spine nice and tall. Hold for 2''.

5. Lastly, fold forward again and repeat this sequence for 5 times.

Note:

This is one of the most advanced stretches in the book, so feel free to skip it if you feel it's too much for you.

It's a dynamic stretch that will open up both the posterior chain and your chest muscles.

CAT COW STRETCH

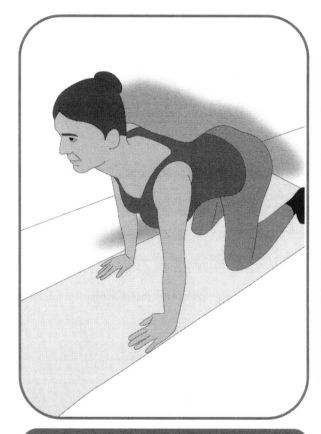

Inhale fully and open up your chest

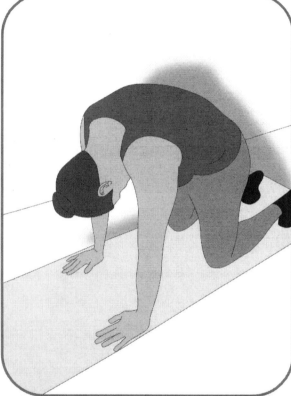

Exhale fully, tuck your chin and bend your spine as comfortably.

How to do it:

1. Start in all four positions with hands below your shoulders and ankles below your knees.

2. From there, inhale fully and open up your chest and look up (as long as it feels comfortable. Hold this stretch for 1-2''.

3. Then. exhale fully via your mouth and arch your upper back until you feel a stretch in the upper-mid back. Bring your chin in as you do so. Hold the stretch for 2''

4. Repeat the sequence for 5 times.

Note:

This is a gentle yet effective stretch to make sure your spine stays healthy and mobile. Often, low back pain is caused by a lack of flexibility in the spine. This exercise will significantly reduce the likelihood of low back pain and feeling of pain and discomfort.

UPPER TRAP RELEASE

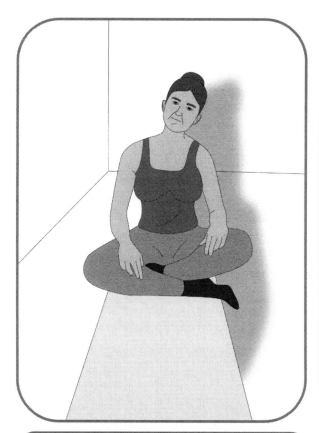

Bend your head to the side towards to your shoulder

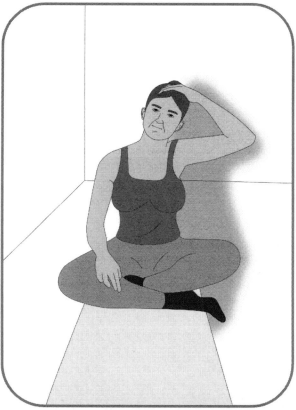

Then, if you feel comfortable, use your hand to apply extra pressure - be sensible

How to do it:

1. Sit on the floor with crossed legs and trunk nice and tall.

2. Bend your head to the side so that your left ear is closer to the left shoulder.

3. Then, push with your left hand your head, so that it gets closer to the left shoulder - do it gently.

4. You will feel a nice stretch on the right side of your neck. hold it for 10'', and then do it on the right side.

Note:

This is a simple yet effective stretch you can also perform sitting or standing.

STANDING EXERCISES

ARM CIRCLING

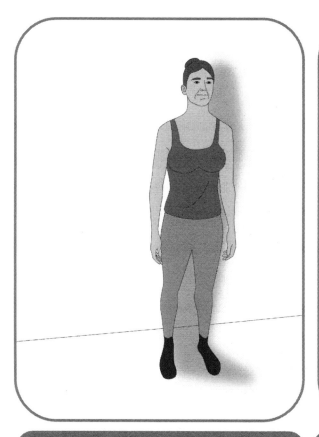

Starting Position – Standing with arms on the side.

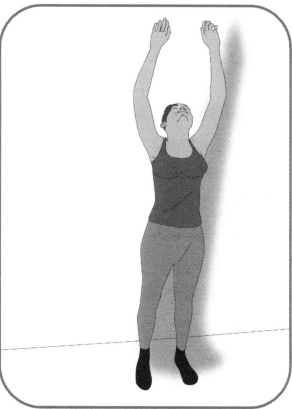

Then, bring your arms up over your head and lift your chin to the ceiling. Repeat for the mentioned reps.

How to do it:

1. Stand tall with feet hip-width apart and arms on the side.

2. Inhale through your nose and bring your arms up. Keep them straight as you do so. As you lift your arms, lift also your chin to the ceiling.

3. Then, always keeping them straight - so perform a semicircle to do it - come back into starting position, and exhale fully. As you do so, come back with the chin in a neutral position.

Note:

In this particular exercise synchronizing the breathing with the arms movement.

TRUNK TWIST

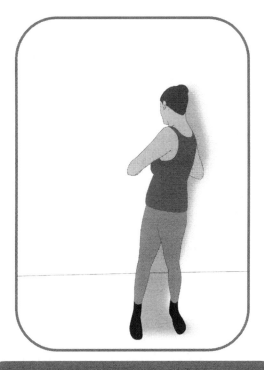

Rotate towards the right side.

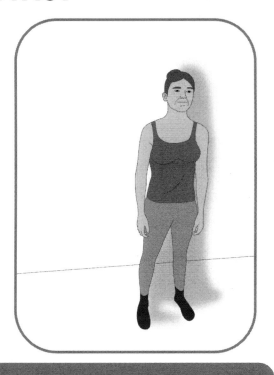

Come back into the starting position

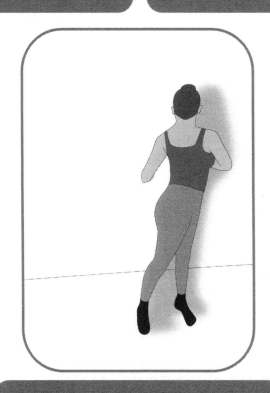

Rotate to the left side

How to do it:

1. Stand with arms on the side and feet hip width apart.

2. From there, rotate towards one side until comfortable. As you rotate, move your head following the trunk, as shown in the image. Hold that position for 1''.

3. Then, come back into the starting position, and repeat on the other side.

Note:

This is a simple stretch to work on the trunk muscles in a way we rarely do. Keeping our rotation movement is very important for daily life activities.

My suggestions are to perform the movement slowly and controlled as well as keeping the stretch for two seconds before coming back into the starting position.

SIDE STRETCH

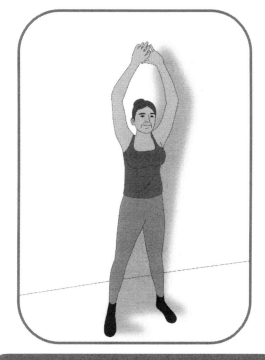

Starting Position - Standing with arms overhead

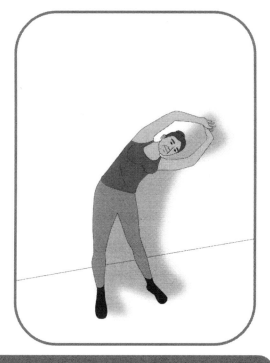

Bend on the left side gently and hold the stretch for 2″

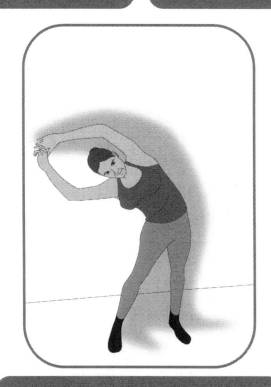

Then, repeat it on the other side.

How to do it:

1. Stand with feet slightly wider than hip-width apart and arms straight over your head.

2. Keep your hands together, and as you exhale bend on one side as much as you feel comfortable. Hold that position for roughly 2''.

3. Then, gently come back into the starting position, and repeat to the other side.

4. Repeat for 5 times on each side.

Note:

One of the most important and effective stretches. My suggestion is to bend as far as you feel comfortable without exaggerating. Overtime I can assure you will be able to go deeper into the stretch which can decrease the likelihood of low back pain and soreness.

To make it easier and avoid losing balance you can spread your legs a slightly wide apart.

CHIN TO THE SKY

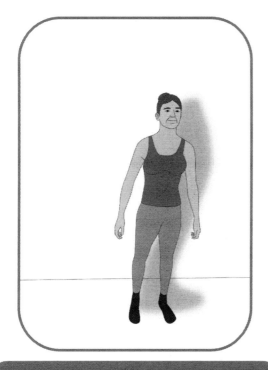

Step 1 - Starting Position

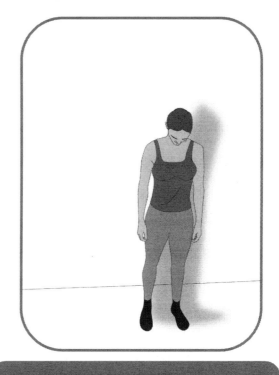

Step 2- Tuck your chin in

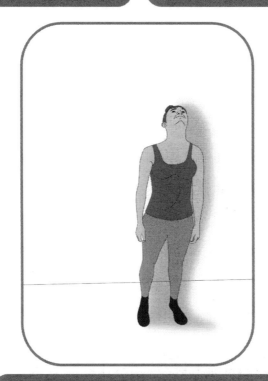

Step 3 - Then, lift your chin as high
as you can. Repeat the sequence

How to do it:

1. Stand with feet hip width apart and hands on the side. Look in front of you.

2. Slowly tuck your chin so that it touches your collarbone (or at least get close to it). Exhale as you do so.

3. Then, gently raise your chin and point it to the sky, tilting your head back. Hold that position for 1''.

4. Repeat 10 times.

Note:

This is going to be useful to tone up the muscles on your neck, preventing loose skin and double chin. It also will improve your neck posture and reduce the risk of forward head which is common due to excessive screen time.

TOE TOUCH + ARM RAISE

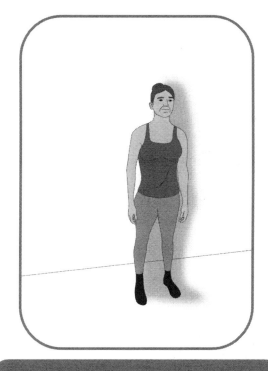

Step 1 - Starting Position

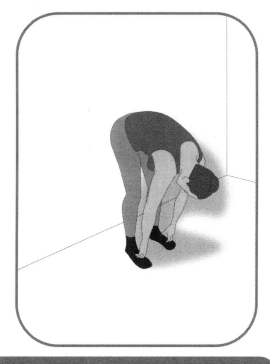

Step 2- Bend your spine and by touching your toes

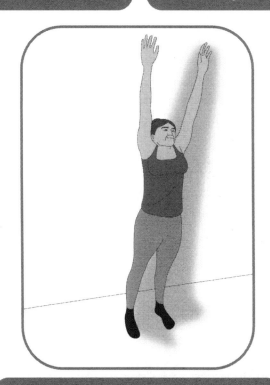

Step 3 - Raise your arms over your head and hold it for 2". Repeat the sequence

How to do it:

1. Stand with feet hip width apart, and arms on the side.

2. From the starting position, bend your spine and try to touch your toes. Hold that position for 1''.

3. Then, come back into the starting position and raise your arms over your head, stretching your spine as much as you can. Hold the stretch for 2''.

4. Repeat the sequence for 5 to 8 times.

Note:

Full body stretch that will awaken as well as relax each part of your body.

Touching your toes is a plus. The idea is that you bend forward as much as you can so that you feel a mild stretch on the back of your leg.

HIP CIRCLE

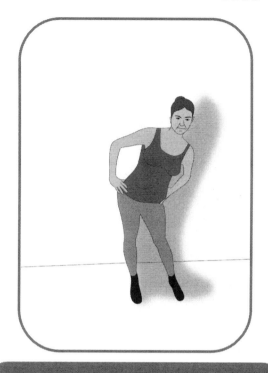

Move your hips in a circle. Going to the right

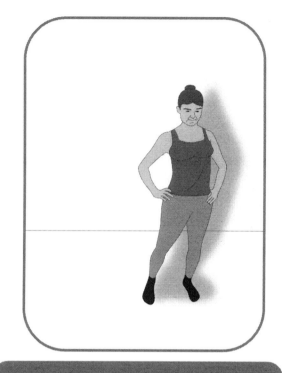

Forward...

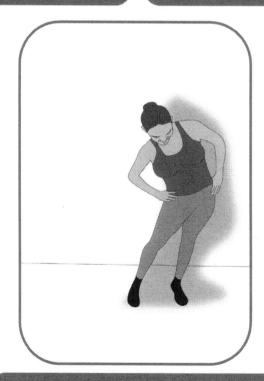

...and to the left. Repeat for the mentioned times

How to do it:

1. Stand with feet hip width apart and hands behind your lower back. Keep your knees slightly bent.

2. From there, move your hips in a circle. Start gently in a clockwise motion. Do it 10 times.

3. Then, move them anticlockwise for 10 times.

Note:

Very gentle exercise to loosen up your waist and get used to this movement. If it feels more comfortable you can position your hands on your waist (one the side, specifically) rather than your lower back.

As an easier alternative, perform Seated Hip Circle (tutorial at page.xx)

HAMSTRING STRETCH

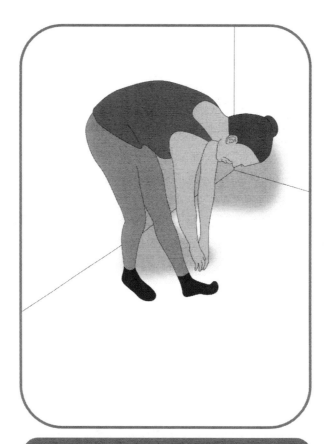

Stretch your left hamstring - Stop when feeling the stretch. Then, do the other leg.

How to do it:

1. From a standing position move one leg straight in front of you with only your heel on the floor (toes up). The back leg is slightly bent.

2. Lean forward and aim to reach for the toes with your arm.

3. Feel the stretch on the back of the leg. Hold it for 10-20'', then repeat it on the other side.

Note:

You do not have to touch your toes. That should be the end goal but there is no need to force the stretch to do that. Simply extend the arm towards your foot and stop once you feel the stretch. This is an amazing stretch especially if you sit for long periods of time and your legs always feel stiff and weak.

If you are very advanced (balance wise too), you could reach for your toes with both arms rather than one arm only. This will make it more challenging both for mobility and balance!

TOE TOUCH

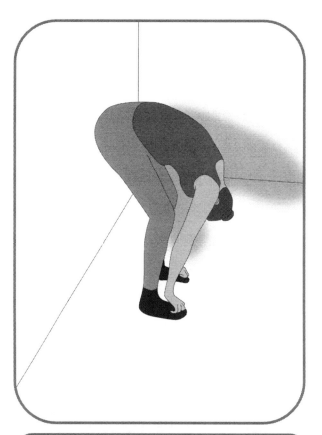

Figure 1 Slide your hands all the way down towards your legs (bending your knee is okay here). Bend your spine as comfortable and feel the stretch for 10-15"

How to do it:

1. Stand with feet hip width apart, arms on the side and knees slightly bent.

2. Place your hands on your thighs, and slide them all the way down until you feel your posterior chain (glutes, back on the thighs and for some people calves too). Hold it for 10-15''. Bending both knees and spine is welcomed in this exercise.

3. Lastly, come back up into the starting position and shake your legs.

Note:

Go all the way down with your arms as far as you can whilst feeling comfortable. Just hang in there.

Once you come up, make sure to do it very slowly, one vertebrae at the time to avoid any discomfort on your back.

HEEL RAISES + ARM SWING

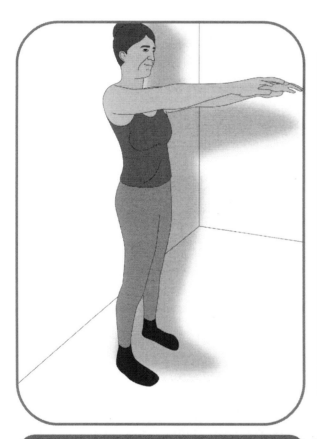

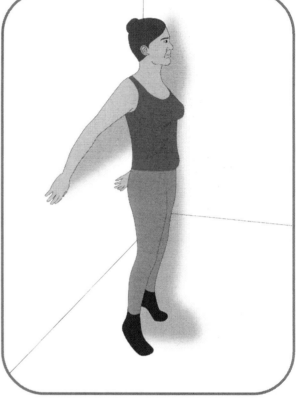

Step 1 - Standing position with arms straight in front of you.

Step 2 - swing arms back and lift your heels as you do so. Then come back into the starting position and repeat for 10 times.

How to do it:

1. Stand with arms straight in front of you and feet hip width apart, as shown in step 1.

2. From there, lift your heels and swing your arms back at the same time.

3. Then, come back into the starting position. Hold 1'' and repeat for 10 times this motion.

Note:

This is one of the most difficult exercises as it requires foot strength, full body coordination and balance.

Do it at your own pace. The faster you do it, the more challenging it will be!

Make sure to keep breathing and not holding your back. At times some people as they entirely focus on mastering the movement "forget" to breathe and tend to hold their breath.

This is something to avoid as it will tense all your body.

BONUS EXERCISE: PLANTAR FASCIA ROLL

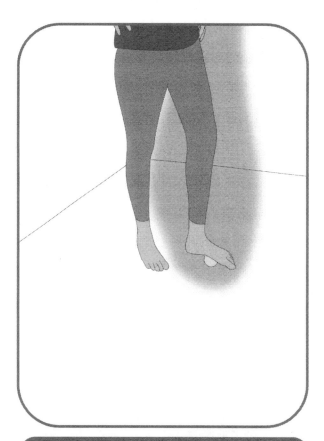

Roll the sole of your foot for anywhere between 2 and 4 minutes

How to do it:

1. Stand and place a tennis ball on your sole. Keep going slowly back and forth on your sole applying a gentle pressure. If you feel any knots or tenderness keep rolling on the area gently to release some pressure

2. Do it for 2-4 minutes each foot.

Note:

This is one of the greatest exercises you can do to relieve stress, decrease anxiety, relieve stress, improve the circulations and lower blood pressure.

This is because rolling a tennis ball on the sole of your foot for anywhere between 3 and 5 minutes is a foot massage that has amazing benefits for your entire body and circulation.

As it will be mentioned at the start of the 4-Week Stretching Plan, I would highly recommend you to do this exercise before every session, for 2-4' for each foot.

4-WEEK PLAN

This plan has been thought to help you get into the stretching position with ease. In fact, you will start with a 3-day per week routine for the first week.

Then, the second will increase up to 4 days per week.

Lastly, the third and fourth will be a 5-day routine.

I would not recommend stretching everyday , unless specific needs to do so, especially for the first month of "stretching exercises". This is because doing too much too soon could be counterproductive.The routine will require only a chair for the seated exercises as well as a mat (ideally, as some exercises will require you to lay down on the floor).

Note: at times it will be mentioned "2 sets of 20'' hold" or "2 sets of 20'' stretch". This means to perform the exercises for 20'', take a small break of 5-10'' and go again.

Also, as we mentioned in the introduction, remember to breathe! It is important that you use this practice to let go of all your physical tension, so breathing relaxingly will help you tremendously.

Everytime there is more than one set it means that you do the exercise, rest for 5-10'' and repeat it (one more time if it is 2 sets, two more times if it is written 3 sets, and so on).

Important: Before starting every session I highly recommend you to do the "Plantar Fascia Roll" Exercises at page.xx

Let's get ready now!

Would you like some more tips to perform the exercises well and effectively? Are you unsure on how to do some exercises and need help?

Contact me at avfitness99coaching@gmail.com or visit my Instagram profile - avfitness99

Looking forward to helping you to maximize your fitness goals!

WEEK 1

Session 1 - Repeat the whole sequence once or twice.

EXERCISE	HOW TO	PAGE
SHOULDER STRETCH	2 sets of 20'' stretch	7
UPPER TRAP RELEASE	1 set of 10''	47
SEATED HIP CIRCLE	10 clockwise + 10 anti-clock-wise	27
KNEELING HAMSTRING STRETCH	1 set of 20'' each side	39
SEATED SPINE STRETCH	1 set of 15''	31
CHIN TO THE SKY	10 times	55

Session 2 - Repeat the whole sequence once or twice.

EXERCISE	HOW TO	PAGE
CHIN TO THE SKY	10 times	55
LUMBAR SPINE STRETCH	1 sets of 30'' stretch	11
HAMSTRING STRETCH	1 set of 15'' each leg	33
CAT COW STRETCH	5 times	45
GLUTE STRETCH	1 set of 15'' each side	37
CHIN TO THE SKY	10 times	55

Session 3 - Repeat the whole sequence once or twice.

EXERCISE	HOW TO	PAGE
LUMBAR ROTATION STRETCH	1 set of 15''' each side	29
TOE TOUCH + ARM RAISE	5 times	57
TRUNK TWIST	5 times on each side	51
GROIN STRETCH	1 set of 20'' each side	13
UPPER TRAP RELEASE	2 sets of 10'' each side	47
HIP CIRCLE	10 times clockwise + 10 times anticlockwise	59

WEEK 2

Session 1- Repeat the whole sequence twice or three times.

EXERCISE	HOW TO	PAGE
KNEELING HAMSTRING STRETCH	1 set of 20'' each side	39
SHOULDER STRETCH (Variation)	2 sets of 20'' hold	9
SEATED SPINE STRETCH	1 set of 20'' each side	31
HIP FLEXOR STRETCH	2 set of 15'' each side	35
CHILD POSE STRETCH	2 sets of 15'' stretch	41

Session 2 - Repeat the whole sequence twice or three times.

EXERCISE	HOW TO	PAGE
TOE TOUCH	2 sets of 15''	63
CHILD POSE STRETCH	2 sets of 15''	41
BACK EXTENSION STRETCH	5 times	43
WRIST FLEXION STRETCH	2 sets of 10'' each side	15
KNEELING HAMSTRING STRETCH	1 set of 20'' each side	39
SIDE STRETCH	1 set of 5 times each side	53

Session 3 - Repeat the whole sequence twice or three times.

EXERCISE	HOW TO	PAGE
HAMSTRING STRETCH	2 sets of 20" each side	33
UPPER TRAP RELEASE	1 set of 10"	47
GLUTE STRETCH	1 set of 15" each side	37
WRIST EXTENSION STRETCH	2 sets of 10" each side	17
BACK EXTENSION STRETCH	2 sets of 5 times	43

Session 4- Repeat the whole sequence twice or three times.

EXERCISE	HOW TO	PAGE
HEEL RAISES + ARM SWING	10 times	65
TOE TOUCH + ARM RAISE	8 times	57
GOAL POST STRETCH	2 sets of 20''	25
PIRIFORMIS STRETCH	2 sets of 10'' each side	19
HAMSTRING STRETCH	1 set of 15'' each side	33

WEEK 3

Session 1 - Repeat the whole sequence three times.

EXERCISE	HOW TO	PAGE
SHOULDER STRETCH	2 sets of 20'' stretch	7
SEATED HIP CIRCLE	10 clockwise + 10 anti-clock-wise	27
TRUNK TWIST	5 times on each side	51
GLUTE STRETCH	2 set of 15'' each side	37
SEATED SPINE STRETCH	1 set of 15'' stretch	31

Session 2 - Repeat the whole sequence three times.

EXERCISE	HOW TO	PAGE
HAMSTRING STRETCH	2 set of 15'' each leg	33
CAT COW STRETCH	5 times	45
CHIN TO THE SKY	10 times	55
LUMBAR SPINE STRETCH	2 sets of 30'' stretch	11
ARM CIRCLING	6 times	49

Session 3 - Repeat the whole sequence three times.

EXERCISE	HOW TO	PAGE
LOWER BODY STRETCH	1 set of 30'' each side	23
TRUNK TWIST	8 times on each side	51
WRIST EXTENSION STRETCH	2 sets of 10''' each side	17
TOE TOUCH	2 sets of 15''	63

Session 4 - Repeat the whole sequence three times.

EXERCISE	HOW TO	PAGE
ARM CIRCLING	6 times	49
GROIN STRETCH	2 sets of 20'' each side	13
HAMSTRING STRETCH	2 sets of 20''	61
LUMBAR ROTATION STRETCH	1 set of 30''' each side	29
BACK EXTENSION STRETCH	2 sets of 5 times	43

Session 5 - Repeat the whole sequence three times.

EXERCISE	HOW TO	PAGE
CALF AND HAMSTRING STRETCH	2 sets of 15'' stretch	21
HEEL RAISES + ARM SWING	10 times	65
CHIN TO THE SKY	10 times	55
SIDE STRETCH	2 sets of 5 times on each side	53
TOE TOUCH + ARM RAISE	6 times	57

WEEK 4

Session 1 - Repeat the whole sequence three times.

EXERCISE	HOW TO	PAGE
WRIST FLEXION STRETCH	2 sets of 10'' each side	15
SEATED SPINE STRETCH	2 set of 20'' each side	31
ARM CIRCLING	6 times	49
CHILD POSE STRETCH	2 sets of 15''	41
HIP FLEXOR STRETCH	2 sets of 15'' each side	35
CHIN TO THE SKY	10 times	55

Session 2 - Repeat the whole sequence three times.

EXERCISE	HOW TO	PAGE
HIP FLEXOR STRETCH	2 set of 15'' each side	35
BACK EXTENSION STRETCH	5 times	43
HIP CIRCLE	10 times clockwise + 10 times anticlockwise	59
SHOULDER STRETCH (Variation)	2 sets of 20'' stretch	9
CHILD POSE STRETCH	2 sets of 15'' stretch	41

Session 3 - Repeat the whole sequence three times.

EXERCISE	HOW TO	PAGE
ARM CIRCLING	6 times	49
CALF AND HAMSTRING STRETCH	2 sets of 15'' stretch	21
TRUNK TWIST	8 times on each side	51
GROIN STRETCH	2 sets of 20'' each side	13

Session 4 - Repeat the whole sequence three times.

EXERCISE	HOW TO	PAGE
SEATED HIP CIRCLE	10 clockwise + 10 anticlock-wise	27
LOWER BODY STRETCH	1 set of 30'' each side	23
HEEL RAISES + ARM SWING	10 times	65
CHILD POSE STRETCH	2 sets of 15''	41

Session 5 - Repeat the whole sequence three times.

EXERCISE	HOW TO	PAGE
PIRIFORMIS STRETCH	2 sets of 10'' each side	19
LUMBAR SPINE STRETCH	2 sets of 30''	11
GOAL POST STRETCH	2 set of 20'' stretch	25
HIP FLEXOR STRETCH	2 set of 15'' each side	35
TRUNK TWIST	8 times on each side	51

Have you finished the 4-Week plan and are you looking to continue your training with a Personalized Plan?

Contact me at avfitness99coaching@gmail.com or visit my Instagram profile - avfitness99

Looking forward to helping you improve even further... this is just the beginning!

CONCLUSION

Thanks for taking the time to learn stretching exercises for seniors to improve your health and well-being. Your commitment to self-care and physical fitness is truly admirable.

This book is full of stretching exercises specifically designed to meet the unique needs of mature bodies. As mentioned previously, feel totally free to contact me in case you are not sure how to perform an exercise or you have other questions related to your fitness.

I can assure you that by diligently incorporating these exercises into your daily routine, you are making a conscious effort to prioritize your health and enhance your quality of life. This will pay off overtime!

Many readers have experienced remarkable improvements in various aspects of their physical well-being after following the 28-day plan presented in this book (or in others I personally wrote, such as "Wall Pilates Workouts for Women", "Wall Pilates for Seniors" or Chair Yoga for Weight Loss".) In this particular program with a focus on stretching, many Individuals who have followed this program have reported the following transformative outcomes:

- **Improved Posture:** Our bodies naturally undergo changes that can impact our posture. However, with regular practice of the targeted stretching exercises outlined in this book, it is possible to restore and maintain proper alignment, which contributes to better posture. In fact, as you have probably experienced, each session comprehends 5-6 exercises that target different areas of your body. By consciously elongating and strengthening the muscles involved in maintaining good posture, you can stand tall and exude confidence.

- **Decreased Back Pain:** Back pain is a common ailment among seniors, often resulting from muscle stiffness, imbalances, or age-related conditions. By incorporating specific stretches that target the muscles supporting the back, such as the hamstrings, hip flexors, and lower back, you can alleviate (and eventually get rid of) tension, increase flexibility, and reduce back pain

- **Injury Reduction, especially after 60:** it is essential to exercise caution to prevent injuries. Regular stretching exercises as the one mentioned play a vital role in injury prevention by improving flexibility, range of motion, and joint stability. By nurturing your body through gentle and purposeful stretches, you can reduce the risk of sprains, strains, and other injuries, ensuring you can continue to enjoy an active and fulfilling life.

Thank you for your dedication to self-improvement and your commitment to your health. By investing in this book and actively participating in the exercises, you are investing in yourself and your future. May your journey be filled with joy, vitality, and a renewed sense of purpose.

Good Luck and Stay Healthy!

ABOUT ME

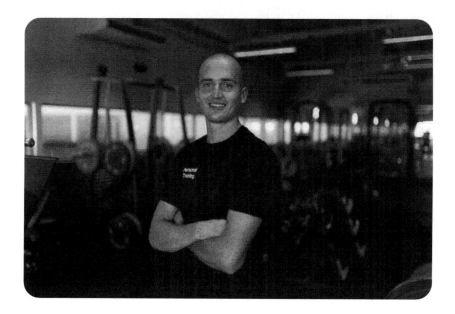

My name is Alessandro...and you might already know me from other books (in that case, hope you have found them useful!)

I am Italian, and I have lived in Milan, London, and Valencia, Spain. My passion for fitness started in my childhood and never stopped since then.

I am a certified Personal Trainer with years of experience in the United Kingdom and Spain. I have been studying fitness articles and guides to make people fitter for years. My experience helping hundreds of people led me to write numerous books on it.

The goal is to make them healthier, more flexible, stronger, and enjoy life more. I have been doing 1-on-1 sessions, group sessions, and online coaching with people of all ages.

I dream of a world in which age is just a number in which everyone is fit regardless of their schedule. With just 10 minutes per day and a good lifestyle people underestimate the results they can get, and this is the message I love to spread across.

Made in United States
Troutdale, OR
10/30/2024

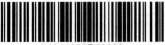